The Miracle of Garlic

Herbal Remedy for Weight Loss, Diabetes, Blood Pressure, Cholesterol, Cancer, Allergies and Much Much More.

David Sykes

Table of Contents

Preview Of 'The Miracle of Green Tea - Herbal Remedy for Weight Loss, Diabetes, Blood Pressure, Cholesterol, Cancer, Allergies and Much, Much More'

Introduction

I want to thank you and congratulate you for purchasing the book, "The Miracle of Garlic: Herbal Remedy for Weight Loss, Diabetes, Blood Pressure, Cholesterol, Cancer, Allergies and Much Much More.".

This book contains proven steps and strategies on how to use garlic in many different ways in order to naturally treat various health conditions. Although garlic is best known as a flavor enhancer added to different kinds of dishes, this herb can be taken or applied using different methods to make the symptoms of your illnesses disappear. Garlic can be taken raw or in supplement form, although making it a staple ingredient in your dishes is the easiest way of reaping its health benefits.

Through this book, you will learn the different ways in which garlic can help you lose weight, manage your diabetes as well as blood pressure and cholesterol levels, and treat or prevent cancer. The book also provides tips on how you can take or prepare garlic in order to cure your allergies, coughs, colds, flu, and other health conditions. Indeed, garlic is such a versatile herbal remedy that is worth keeping in your arsenal of natural treatments.

Thanks again for purchasing this book, I hope you enjoy it!

Chapter 1 Getting to Know Garlic

Originating from central Asia, garlic is a perennial plant that is now grown in many parts of the world, reaching heights of two or more feet. The part of garlic which is used as remedy is its compound bulb, each of which consists of four to twenty cloves. Supplements from garlic can be made in various forms – fresh, aged, dried, or oil-based, with each form affecting the body in a different way.

World-Renowned Herb

Garlic is now being recognized by experts in modern medicine for its effectiveness and numerous health benefits. But garlic has been used for over 3,000 years in different parts of the world for treatment as well as prevention of various health conditions.

Nature's Medicine Chest

Numerous studies have shown that garlic is like nature's medicine chest, containing over 400 chemical components at last count. Most of these chemical components are released through chewing or crushing raw garlic to induce the breakdown of allicin. Garlic also contains sulfur compounds which have been identified as a powerful killer of bacteria, fungi, viruses, and parasites.

Powerful Health Aid

Other chemical compounds of garlic also work hand in hand with vital systems in your body, including your immunological, digestive, and circulatory systems. The results – cleansing, detoxification, healing, and strengthening – provide garlic the ability to promote overall good health.

Multitasking Herbal Remedy

The list of things that garlic is able to do to benefit your health only further cements its fame as a multitasking herbal remedy. It effectively strengthens your immune system, acts as an antioxidant, and even functions as a detoxifying agent. Garlic also has the ability to thin your blood, as well as reduce your blood cholesterol and blood sugar levels. Furthermore, it has the potential to fight diseases affecting your respiratory system, as well as cancer, herpes, and HIV/AIDS infections.

Promising Treatment for Dreaded Diseases

It has been determined that garlic shows great potential in terms of treating a number of dreaded diseases today, which include HIV infections, breast cancer, and coronary heart disease. Moreover, a number of major conventional antibiotics have found their competition in garlic in terms of effectively eliminating potentially dangerous strains of bacteria like Staphylococcus and Streptococcus, which are now showing greater resistance to many antibiotics made in the laboratory.

Wonder Drug

What is remarkable about garlic is that, while Enterococcus, Staphylococcus, Streptococcus, and other harmful bacteria tend to resist tetracycline, penicillin, vancomycin, and other conventional antibiotics, they do not have the ability to develop a resistance to garlic. Moreover, garlic does not destroy the beneficial bacteria in your intestines, which is what conventional antibiotics do.

Available in Various Forms

Whole fresh garlic, dried or freeze-dried garlic, aged garlic extracts, and garlic oil are utilized in order to make garlic supplements. Because different forms of garlic have different amounts of active ingredients, it is crucial to read garlic supplement labels with care. Standardized garlic products are your best bet if you want to get the most out of your garlic supplements. It is also important to consult and follow the advice of a healthcare provider or an herbal medicine expert regarding the proper use of garlic supplements.

Biologically Active

Promoting health as well as treating various illnesses with the use of garlic and other herbs is an approach that has long been practiced. This does not disregard the fact, however, that herbs have the potential to cause side effects as well as detrimental interactions with other herbs, medications, or supplements. This is the reason why it is important to take herbs with the guidance of a healthcare provider who is knowledgeable on plant medicine.

Side Effects. Handling large amounts of fresh or dried garlic can cause a stinging sensation or a lesion to occur on your skin. Taking garlic supplements may also lead to bloating, stomach upset, body odor, and bad breath. You may also experience other uncommon side effects of taking garlic supplements, such as muscle aches, fatigue, headache, dizziness, loss of appetite, skin rash, and asthma. Taking too much garlic, which has the ability to cause thinning of the blood, can also cause you to bleed while undergoing surgery or after. It is also important to seek your doctor's advice if you happen to have a thyroid problem or an ulcer.

Possible Interactions. Garlic can potentially interact with a number of prescription medicines you may be taking, especially those intended for blood-thinning. Be safe by asking your doctor's advice before deciding to take garlic supplements.

Chapter 2 Miraculous Health Benefits of Garlic for Weight Loss, Diabetes, Blood Pressure, Cholesterol, Cancer, and Allergies

Recognized as one of the most potent herbal remedies in the world, the health benefits as well as the effectiveness of garlic are comparable to those offered by modern medicines.

Weight Loss

Why Garlic is an Effective Herbal Remedy for Weight Loss

Garlic has anti-obesity properties that make it an effective aid in losing excess weight. In fact, this herb has been identified in studies to have the ability to slow down your body's adipogenesis, or the process of producing fat cells. Besides eating it raw, making garlic a staple in your diet is, therefore, also a great way of ensuring that you do not easily gain weight.

How to Use Garlic for Weight Loss

The manner in which garlic is prepared greatly affects its power to act as an herbal remedy. It is important to let garlic sit for about ten minutes after mashing, slicing, or chopping its cloves. The garlic cloves should also be kept away from heat while letting them sit. This way, they are exposed to the air, allowing garlic's active substance allicin to be formed. What is great about allicin is that it does not break down even when garlic is cooked.

Diabetes

Why Garlic is an Effective Herbal Remedy for Diabetes

The sweet surprise of garlic is that it has the ability to regulate your blood sugar levels by increasing the amount of insulin produced in your body, which is why it makes such a great addition to your diet and to your arsenal of natural remedies for diabetes. Garlic can never replace insulin or other diabetes medications, but eating it raw as well as making it a part of your diet may decrease your need for additional insulin.

How to Use Garlic for Diabetes

Garlic can be added to dishes prepared in various ways. The important thing to remember is to activate its allicin component before cooking.

Blood Pressure and Cholesterol

Why Garlic is an Effective Herbal Remedy for Blood Pressure and Cholesterol

Studies have documented the positive effect that garlic has on your blood pressure and cholesterol level. This herb has been proven to lower your blood pressure (by causing your vein and artery walls to relax), lower the amount of your bad cholesterol, and increase your good cholesterol levels. Because of these actions, garlic has the ability to protect you from having a heart attack or a stroke.

How to Use Garlic for Blood Pressure and Cholesterol

1. Eat Raw Cloves

Aim to buy the freshest garlic bulbs that you possibly can. If available, it would be better if you are able to score organic ones. Because the peels can harbor mold or bacteria, always peel them off and wash the garlic cloves well before swallowing them with some drinking water.

Research has demonstrated that risks for succeeding heart attacks have been reduced to half when patients took 2 to 3 cloves of garlic daily. This sounds hopeful, but the fact that you will come off smelling like garlic if you eat it is unfortunate. Fortunately, there are ways you can freshen your breath while reaping the benefits of taking garlic, including chewing on a cinnamon stick, eating fresh parsley or mint, and drinking lemon juice or water.

2. Take a Capsule

If you truly cannot stand the taste or smell of garlic, you could always opt to take it in capsules, extracts, or tablets instead. Extracts of aged garlic that you can get in health food stores are your best bet. Studies have indicated that one garlic capsule daily – taken during your main meal and with a cold beverage – contains just the right amount of allicin that promotes overall good health and wellbeing. It is important to check the dosage in different brands; some may require you to take as much as three to five capsules per day.

3. Drink a Garlic-Infused Beverage

A garlic-infused beverage is easy to make. Simply place two teaspoons of powdered garlic and two cups of boiling water in a ceramic pot (although a stainless steel or glass version works just as well). Stir continuously to dissolve the powder well. Cover the teapot and allow the concoction to sit for about ten minutes before drinking it.

4. Add to Foods

Various dishes include garlic in their list of ingredients because of the distinctive aroma and flavor it imparts, especially when used with other herbs such as onion and ginger. The method of cooking used will determine if the flavor of garlic turns out intense or mellow, depending on your preference.

Cancer

Why Garlic is an Effective Herbal Remedy for Cancer

Since the ancient times, garlic has been recognized for its ability to heal a number of health conditions. With new evidence that it can be used to effectively fight cancer, garlic is now being put on the spotlight again by the medical community. Scientists have determined that the large amounts of sulfides contained in garlic give the herb the ability to prevent tumors from flourishing, as well as to reduce the activity of cancer-causing agents. Garlic has been identified by experts in cancer research as among the top foods to eat to protect oneself from a number of forms of cancer.

Add the fact that garlic is abundant in antioxidants, which makes the herb potent against cancer. But it is important to keep in mind that garlic is best taken either raw or cooked since supplements do not appear to have a similar cancer-fighting effect.

How to Use Garlic for Cancer

Use garlic as a natural flavor enhancer in various dishes – this is the easiest way for you to make use of garlic's miraculous cancer-healing power.

By the way, these groups of anti-cancer food are most potent against the dreaded disease: cruciferous vegetables, green tea, omega 3 essential fatty acids, olive oil, tomatoes, garlic and onions, soy products, berries and citrus fruits, as well as red wine and dark chocolate.

Allergies

Why Garlic is an Effective Herbal Remedy for Allergies

People usually don't have an idea what to do when their allergies hit them, when they have an infection, or when they catch an illness. What makes it even more difficult is that more and more individuals are beginning to lose faith in medications as well as in the doctors who prescribe them. This prompts many to turn to other drugs which either do not do anything or potentially cause harm.

This is where garlic comes in as a great herbal remedy to use when treating allergies. Garlic naturally has antibiotic properties that do not kill off healthy bacteria in the process, which is what antibiotic drugs do. Moreover, garlic oil has expectorant and decongestant qualities. Garlic is also a potent cold treatment since it contains vitamin C, certain enzymes, selenium, sulfur, and other minerals.

Chapter 3 Powerful Health Benefits of Garlic for the Immune System

It is not surprising that the high amounts of antioxidants present in garlic give it the ability to improve your immune system, protecting your body from the attacks of all forms of bacteria and virus. Garlic has also been shown to be an effective cold remedy, decongestant, and expectorant. With its abundant amounts of vitamins C and B6, as well as selenium, manganese, and other important minerals, garlic has traditionally been linked to boosting the immune system and other health benefits.

Powerful Antibiotic

Garlic is not only effective as an immune system booster and disease fighter. It is also a powerful killer of a wide array of microbes which cause the common cold and other similar ailments. As mentioned earlier, garlic has been studied by researchers for its components, of which at least four hundred have been identified. Out of those numerous chemical components, researchers have singled out allicin, allyl methyl thiosulfinate, diallyl trisulfide, and ajoene as the powerful substances that give garlic its antibiotic properties.

A number of conventional antibiotics have been found to be nowhere as effective as garlic, and may even cause the destruction of good intestinal flora. Studies have also shown that after a long time of repeated use, antibiotics that are manufactured in the laboratory may lose their effectiveness once a bacteria strain becomes resistant to them. Fortunately, this is not the case with garlic, because bacteria or even viruses are not able to develop resistance to it. Moreover, intestinal flora is not destroyed when you take garlic in the amounts prescribed to you by your doctor.

You will benefit from using garlic regularly, whether as a supplement, as an addition to soups, stews, salads, and juices, or as treatment for flu, a cold, or sore throat. When taking garlic, and especially when you are ill, it is important to avoid any form of caffeine, alcohol, and sugar, which all cause your immunity to dip.

Effective Stress and Fatigue Fighter

Because garlic also acts as a restorative herb, it has the ability to promote balance in a stress-filled life and overly tired body. It is already such a great relief to know that garlic can give us protection against hypertension, high blood pressure, and other diseases. But it is also good to know that garlic works as an effective tonic to help reduce your fatigue and other stress symptoms. Moreover, garlic has the ability to elevate your energy levels, give your physical stamina a boost, and lengthen your lifespan.

Using garlic as a tonic has already been practiced during the ancient times. In fact, instances of Egyptians providing garlic tonics to their slaves for them to be able to resist illnesses and reduce their tiredness, have been noted in historical records. Whenever the Egyptians failed to do so due to shortage, the slaves reportedly rose in rebellion against them.

Key Player against HIV Infections

The immune system is easily weakened when attacked by HIV, presenting an opportunity for various diseases to set in. Garlic helps by boosting your immune system and killing off various invading microorganisms such as viruses, bacteria, and fungi in the process. Moreover, garlic is actually recommended by a number of practitioners of alternative medicine, in addition to a nutrient or medical program they prescribe. They have found that garlic is effective in protecting the body from infections when used as food.

Garlic has also been found by researchers to have the potential to act against Herpes, Cryptococcus, Cytomegalovirus, Pneumocystis, Mycobacteria, Cryptosporidia, and other common infection-causing microbes associated with AIDS. This shows that garlic may have the ability to stop the proliferation of HIV in an AIDS patient.

So far, what has been determined is that garlic is able to activate three types of cells involved with the immune system, each of which has a role in fighting off HIV and AIDS-associated infections. It has been found that one of garlic's powerful compounds, diallyl trisulfide, can actually set various natural killer cells in motion, including the phagocytes (which have the ability to swallow invading germs), the cytotoxic T-cells (which work by getting themselves attached to microbes and then secreting their poisonous substances into the latter), and the lymphocytes (which kill specific microorganisms with the antibodies they make).

Chapter 4 Herbal Remedies Using Garlic (Part I)

Treatment for Itchy, Sore Throat

You don't have to suffer in misery from having an itchy, sore throat due to a flu virus or a common cold you caught, or because you were infected with strep or staph. Garlic can help you get well and get out of being trapped in bed for several days. You can easily make an anti-itch-sore remedy for your throat and use it to treat your condition, especially if your throat irritation is not caused by acid reflux, an allergy, a tumor, or any other more serious or chronic health condition.

Before the itch you feel at the back of your throat gets any worse, work on it immediately with the use of garlic. You may crush one raw garlic clove and spread it onto your favorite piece of bread. Drizzle with some olive oil or any cooking oil (plain) and then sprinkle a pinch of salt. Chew the bread and then gradually swallow. The itch in your throat will almost instantly go away, although you may still have to repeat the process in order to kill off any germs left lurking.

While it is true that a cough drop or an herbal lozenge (especially if it contains eucalyptus, peppermint, sage, anise, or fennel) does help to soothe an itchy, sore throat, garlic works better because it does not only eliminate the irritation – it also kills off the culprit behind it.

Treatment for Acne

Garlic may not be a staple in your medication stash for acne, but it actually makes an effective natural remedy for acne-related issues such as unwanted skin blemishes. The reason for its effectiveness lies in its antioxidant properties. Treat your acne by simply rubbing a sliced garlic clove on the affected area.

Garlic works in treating acne issues because, as researchers have found out, it actually contains a powerful antioxidant that is more potent than those of oranges, papayas, or any other food. It has been reported in a study made on the power of garlic as an herbal remedy that allicin does not merely provide the herb its unique flavor and odor, but that it is also able to break down into sulfenic acid, which is considered the ultimate antioxidant. It has been said that the fast reaction of sulfenic acid and harmful radicals upon contact is the reason for garlic's ability to treat acne.

Using garlic in acne treatment is not difficult. You simply have to make sure that you consume the garlic in its raw form to get the most benefit. Crush some garlic cloves and then add to your meals. You might try complementing your Italian pasta with some garlic bread, for example. To effectively prevent acne, consuming a couple of garlic cloves daily is recommended. It would also be best to take garlic fresh, since the level of antioxidants in garlic is highest when it is still fresh.

You might also want to try making your own homemade topical remedy for acne. Get one clove of garlic and crush it thoroughly until a paste is made. Add about one-half cup of warm water to dilute the garlic paste. Using a clean washcloth, apply the paste to your face. Afterwards, use a mild cleanser to wash it off. Because the mixture is diluted with water, you do not have to worry about experiencing any irritation, although you should immediately stop the treatment if you experience any burning sensation.

Treatment for Allergies

1. Drink Garlic Milk for Asthma

Warm garlic milk is a natural asthma remedy you can try, especially if you are a believer of traditional medicine. Prepare garlic milk by simply mashing eight pieces of raw garlic cloves (with their skins peeled off) and then placing them in a medium ceramic pot. Take ¼ cup of fresh organic milk and pour into the pot. Over low heat, bring the garlic and milk mixture to a gentle boil. Use a wooden spatula to stir continuously and prevent milk solids from being formed. After about five minutes, remove the pot from the heat and remove the garlic from the heated mixture by straining. Let the milk cool down a bit before drinking it.

2. Rub Sliced Raw Garlic on Insect Bite Allergy

Insect sting allergies can easily be treated with the use of raw garlic. Just take one garlic clove, slice it in half, and then rub the juicy portion on the insect bite. This treatment is particularly helpful if the bite has already developed a slight infection.

3. Apply Garlic Compress on Skin Allergies

Skin allergies should not be a problem when help from a garlic compress is on the way. Just place two teaspoons of crushed garlic in a small saucepan and add two cups of water. Bring the mixture to a boil over medium heat, after which you should cover the saucepan and reduce the heat to low. Allow the mixture to simmer for about fifteen minutes before turning off the heat. Once cooled, take a clean linen cloth and soak in the garlic decoction. Place the garlic compress on your affected skin; it helps if you keep the compress warm with a hot water bottle placed above it.

Treatment for Respiratory Illnesses

1. Drink Garlic Syrup for Coughs

To make your garlic cough syrup, peel the skins off about 25 to 30 garlic cloves (equal to an entire head of garlic). Place in a small mixing bowl, and then add raw apple cider vinegar (1/4 cup), water (1/2 cup), and raw honey (1/2 cup). Make sure the wet ingredients completely cover the garlic cloves. Let the mixture sit overnight before straining the pulp. Store your garlic syrup in a dark, airtight bottle and keep it in a place that is cool and dry. Treat your cough by taking a teaspoon every two hours until your symptoms disappear.

2. Take Honey and Garlic for Colds

Treat your cold symptoms by taking one head of garlic, breaking up the cloves, peeling the skins off, and mincing and mashing them all together in a small bowl. Pour one-half cup of raw honey over the mashed garlic, and then stir well to until you achieve a thick consistency. Let the honey and garlic paste sit for about five minutes before stirring it again. Take a teaspoonful of this paste regularly to clear your cold and completely relieve its symptoms.

3. Drink Orange Juice with Garlic for Flu

Peel the skin off one garlic clove and cut into thin slices. Let the garlic slices sit for about ten to fifteen minutes. Take one teaspoon of the garlic slices and swallow with the help of one glassful of orange juice. This flu treatment works best when done right before your bedtime at night. Make sure to repeat the process until your flu goes away.

Chapter 5 Herbal Remedies Using Garlic (Part II)

Garlic may be taken in different forms, as well as applied topically using different preparations, to treat a number of health conditions.

Amoebic Dysentery

Going on a trip abroad (especially to a third world country) can cause you to have diarrhea or some form of stomach upset referred to as amoebic dysentery. Bacteria or parasites that are present in local drinking water are the reason for your getting amoebic dysentery. For several times a day, take either raw garlic cloves or garlic capsules to kill any microbe that has found its way inside your body and treat your stomach condition.

Arthritis

Whether in raw or capsule form, garlic has an excellent anti-inflammatory property when taken every day. This gives garlic the ability to provide pain relief from arthritis.

Athlete's Foot

Besides being anti-inflammatory by nature, garlic is also anti-bacterial, making it a good remedy for athlete's foot. To get rid of the fungus, as well as relieve you of inflammation, you can do any of the following:

- Use garlic juice to cleanse your feet.
- Apply crushed or powdered garlic directly on the affected area, leaving it on for two minutes before rinsing off.
- Eat cooked or raw garlic on a daily basis for prevention.

Boils

To draw the boils out and make it easy for you to drain them with a sterile needle, it helps to apply garlic poultice on them. (You can easily make a garlic poultice by simply crushing some raw garlic, placing it directly on your boils, and then covering it with a clean bandage or cloth.) Fresh poultice should then be reapplied until the boils are healed. To enable the poultice to penetrate the boils more, try using a hot water bottle to warm it up.

Candida/Yeast Infection

Garlic naturally has antifungal properties that enable it to eliminate yeast. You can reduce your yeast infection by taking garlic capsules or raw garlic cloves on a daily basis. Also, taking garlic seems to increase the potency of a Candida diet plan you might be following or any yeast infection supplements you may be taking.

Ear Infection

Try placing a couple of drops of garlic oil into your affected ear, and then inserting a cotton ball to keep the oil in. You should do this several times daily until your ear infection heals. (To make garlic oil, blend ½ cup of minced fresh garlic and ½ cup of olive oil thoroughly. Add an additional ¼ cup of olive oil before stirring the mixture. Place in a sealed glass container. Let the mixture sit for ten days in a sunny area of your house, making sure to shake the jar thrice a day. Strain the mixture at the end of the 10-day period, transfer the garlic oil into a tightly-sealed glass jar, and store in the refrigerator.)

Ringworm

Due to its antifungal property, garlic is an effective herbal remedy for fungal infections such as ringworm. Just take a few peeled garlic cloves and cut them into thin slices. Place on the ringworm-infected area and cover with gauze. Leave the gauze on overnight and remove the morning after. Repeat the process even after the ringworm infection heals to prevent the spread of ringworm to other areas.

Skin Infection

Garlic's antibacterial qualities enable it to effectively work as an herbal remedy, both internally and externally. You can dust some garlic powder on your infected skin and either cover it up with bandage or just leave it as is. You may also mix garlic powder and coconut oil, which acts effectively as an antibacterial and antifungal agent itself, to create a cream you can rub on the skin infection.

Thrush

Adults who have a thrush infection can simply chew raw garlic cloves to overcome it. Well, you could also take garlic capsules to help clear the yeast overgrowth inside your mouth. If it is your baby who has a thrush infection, give him a small dose of garlic oil instead. An infant could use just one drop of garlic oil, while two drops may be needed by a young child.

Warts

Take a slice of raw garlic. Place the wet side down on your wart and then cover with a small bandage. Replace the garlic slice and bandage every morning and night until your wart disappears. It helps if you leave the treatment on overnight. You may notice that the size of your wart becomes reduced, although black marks (small dots) may be left on the affected skin. Repeat this treatment until the black dots disappear.

Wounds

Crush a couple of raw garlic cloves in a small mixing bowl. Add one cup of water and mix well. Use this mixture to wash your open wound. Then take one-half teaspoon of garlic powder and apply directly on your wound. To speed up the healing process, as well as prevent infection, it helps to apply some dressing on the wound. (It would still be ideal to wash the wound before applying garlic in any form, as doing so ensures that disease-causing microbes are kept at a minimum. Moreover, if the wound seems too painful or too wide, it might be best to simply rush to the emergency room instead of applying any kind of herbal remedy. As a final reminder, don't forget that the concentration of garlic affects how much pain it will cause upon application – if you're the kind who's rather sensitive to pain, you may want to consider an alternative.)

Conclusion

Thank you again for purchasing this book!

I hope this book was able to help you learn about the numerous ways that garlic can be used to treat different health conditions.

The next step is to take into consideration that as much as garlic helps you as an herbal remedy, you have to watch out for potential side effects (such as upset stomach, headache, muscle aches, fatigue, dizziness, loss of appetite, or heartburn) and possible interactions (allergic reactions such as eczema) with other herbal remedies, medications, or supplements. It is important that you seek advice from a healthcare provider, especially one who has extensive knowledge in herbal medicine.

The most common complaint against garlic, which is the reason many people may be hesitant to use it as an herbal remedy, is that it leaves a distinct odor that they may find unpleasant. But drinking lemon juice, sipping lemon water, or eating lemon slices can help a lot in preventing garlic breath.

Garlic is also known to cause thinning of the blood. If you have a history of a blood disorder, have a surgical operation scheduled, or are about to deliver a baby, it would be wise to do away with taking fresh garlic or garlic supplements. It is also best to refrain from using garlic as an herbal remedy if you have an ulcer or gastroenteritis, and if you are pregnant or are nursing.

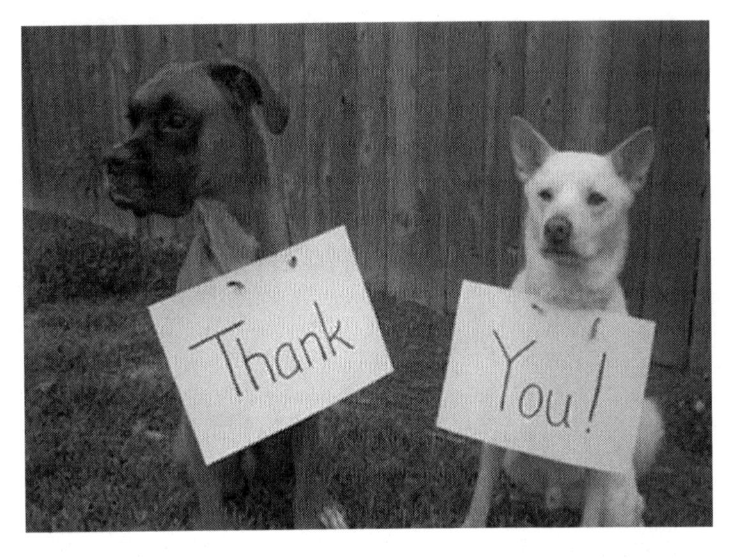

Finally, if you enjoyed this book, then I'd like to ask you for a favor, would you be kind enough to leave a review for this book on Amazon? It'd be greatly appreciated!

Thank you and good luck!

Preview Of 'The Miracle of Green Tea - Herbal Remedy for Weight Loss, Diabetes, Blood Pressure, Cholesterol, Cancer, Allergies and Much, Much More'

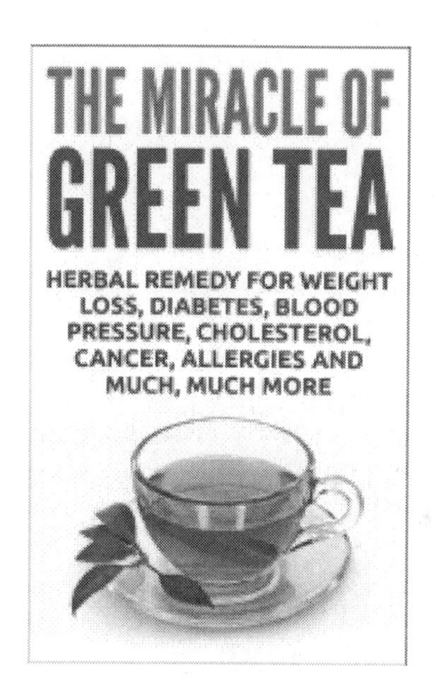

Chapter 1 - The Tea as You Know It

In Asia and Europe, locals from the ancient and contemporary times enjoy a cup of green tea. This brew from the *Camellia sinensis* plant originated from China, and was also transported to India and other parts of the world. Even now, green tea is revered as a super drink because of the following benefits:

- Prevents cancer
- Helps regulate cholesterol levels
- Controls blood pressure
- Strengthens the immune system
- Suppresses the growth of tumors
- Reduces the chances of stroke and epilepsy
- Manages blood sugar levels
- Slows down the aging process

It is also astonishing that the Japanese, who drink green tea every day, have longer life spans than most Americans and Europeans. The Japanese's vegan diet helps, but green tea should also be accounted for their good health and long life. In fact, green tea has been considered a medicine in China for 4,000 years and was even called the "divine elixir of the gods". Why wouldn't it be, when it can do a lot of things and its efficacy has been proven by physicians and scientists?

As an evergreen shrub, *Camellia sinensis* grows with fragrant blooms. To reproduce, this plant must be cross-pollinated with another tea plant. They are also not genetically modified; they are grown with care until the leaves are ready for plucking. Even the plucking is done by hands, never by machines, because it could crush or rip off the leaves and results to fermentation – definitely a no-no in the production of tea.

The plucked leaves will then be subjected to processing. They are processed through any of the following means: steaming, withering, drying, rolling, or a combination of these processes. Green tea, specifically, is prepared in these ways: First, it will be steamed after harvesting the leaves. Steaming (some people use the term 'pan-firing') makes the leaves pliable and soft. Next, the leaves will be rolled to lessen the moisture content. The leaves will also be twisted and dried.

The process is done carefully so that the leaves do not lose polyphenols. These are potent health boosters that are present in vegetables and fruits. Their sub-category – catechins – are also powerful antioxidants. To keep the polyphenols in the green tea, the leaves must be pan-fired over charcoal or wood, steamed for about 20-50 seconds, or rotated in heated cylinders for not more than 10 minutes.

Green tea also contains the following:

- Vitamin E that helps slow down aging
- Flavonols that destroy free radicals
- Flouride that prevents the onset of cavities
- Vitamin C that fights stress and infection
- Vitamin B complex that helps in the digestion and metabolism of carbohydrates

Truly, these health promoters make green tea one of the essential beverages in your kitchen. Just imagine loading your system with catechins and these vitamins! You also enjoy the scent of tea, which has a sort of spicy aroma to it. This is why drinking tea is said to have a calming effect – it also caters to all your senses.

If you are interested in buying this book, please

go to: http://amzn.to/1lAOMkB or search for the title "The Miracle of Green Tea"

Thanks You!

David Sykes.

Made in the USA
Las Vegas, NV
05 February 2022